HOW GARLIC PROTECTS YOUR HEART

by E Ernst MD PhD

Published by
Amberwood Publishing Ltd
Park Corner, Park Horsley, East Horsley, Surrey KT24 5RZ
Tel: 01483 285919

First Edition January 1996

ISBN 1-899308-08-3

Typeset and designed by
Word Perfect, Christchurch, Dorset.

Cover design by Design Hive

Printed in Great Britain

PLANTLIFE

The Natural History Museum, Cromwell Road, London SW7 5BD

Registered Charity No. 328576

Amberwood Publishing supports the Plantlife Charity,
Britain's only charity exclusively dedicated to saving wild plants.

CONTENTS

About the Author

Professor Edzard Ernst qualified as a doctor of medicine from Ludwig Maximilian Universität in Munich in 1976. After completing his MD and PhD theses he continued to specialise in Physical Medicine and Rehabilitation. In addition to Professorships at the Universities of Hanover and Vienna he is currently the Professor in Complementary Medicine at the University of Exeter, the first and only chair in this field in Britain. The focus of the chair's research is the efficacy, safety and cost of complementary therapies. Professor Ernst's eminent and prolific career has encompassed a broad range of research from cardiovascular to psychiatric. It has included more than 700 publications, including around 150 original papers, the first paper concerning the medicinal properties of Garlic having been published in 1981. He is the founder of two medical journals and has written and edited eighteen medical books. Professor Ernst's work has resulted in eight prizes for scientific merit between 1984 and 1991.

Preface

An old truism in medicine claims that prevention is better than cure. No question, if we could prevent a meaningful amount of illness we would make savings both in human suffering as well as in health related costs. The overall objective of prevention is to reduce the risk of falling ill and thereby lower disease and death rates and prolong survival.

Considering its relative youth, preventative medicine has already made significant progress which can be translated into "real life" and significantly contributes to preventing premature deaths. Most notably perhaps the progress lies in the field of cardiovascular diseases.

During the past decades a marked increase in the frequency of heart disease and subsequent deaths has been recorded. In most industrialised countries, the death rate due to heart disease has now either stopped increasing or has actually decreased. Yet most of us would like to see much more progress and ask, why are things so slow? The simple but undoubtedly correct answer is, because "things" invariably are very complex. To prevent a disease like coronary heart disease, one has to first understand its causes and its natural course. Subsequently one might decide that prevention is a possibility and try to identify an intervention that could lead to the desired result. This preventive intervention has then to be tested – just as we today demand a therapy to be of proven efficacy, a preventive intervention has to be demonstrated to work. Amongst others we need to know the size of the effect it brings about, how safe the intervention is and how much it costs. Once all this is properly evaluated, we have to design a strategy so as to best translate our knowledge into effective action.

Quite obviously, such research requires time, know-how and money. In the case of heart disease, it has taken some five decades to arrive where we are today, where many heart attacks and strokes can be prevented. This book will look at some aspects of the prevention of coronary heart disease and will detail our present knowledge about the beneficial effects which *Garlic* may have in this respect.

Note to Reader

Whilst the author has made every effort to ensure that the contents of this book are accurate in every particular, it is not intended to be regarded as a substitute for professional medical advice under treatment. The reader is urged to give careful consideration to any difficulties which he or she is experiencing with their own health and to consult their General Practitioner if uncertain as to its cause or nature. Neither the author nor the publisher can accept any legal responsibility for any health problem which results from use of the self-help methods described.

1 | The heart and the circulation of blood

To understand the influence of garlic, we need to comprehend how our body's circulatory system works. The heart is basically a muscle that forms a mechanical pump. Unlike other muscles it is not under voluntary control but functions "automatically", without us noticing. It pumps blood into our lungs where the red blood cells take up some of the oxygen that we breathe in. The oxygen-rich blood is then returned to the heart and circulated to every single organ and (with only very few exceptions) to every body tissue. It flows through big arteries into smaller and smaller ones. In the most tiny capillaries the oxygen is extracted and used up by the tissues. The tissue cells need oxygen to function; without it they would die off quickly. The oxygen-poor blood is subsequently drawn back to the heart through the veins, and the cycle of oxygenation and de-oxygenation starts over again. Therefore our blood can be seen as the transport vehicle (mainly) for oxygen which is carried along the big transport lines, the blood vessels (arteries and veins). The energy to drive it around its circular pathways is supplied by the heart. Blood must never stop flowing and this is why the heart has to carry on pumping incessantly as long as we live.

Without oxygen our organs, which are composed of many cells, would virtually starve to death. If the heart ever stopped, we would be dead within minutes. The heart is therefore a most amazing organ – all other muscles get tired and must rest frequently, but the heart just never does. It is obvious that it needs a constant supply of energy.

Like (almost) all other tissues, the heart is supplied with arteries – in this case the coronary arteries. These are connected to essentially the same circuit as all the other blood vessels of the body. The pumping action of the heart thus guarantees the heart's own supply of oxygen and other sources of energy.

2 | Coronary heart disease

When you feel your own pulse, you actually sense how the heart pumps blood through the arteries. Each contraction of the heart muscle leads to a wave of blood shooting into the periphery. This creates regular waves of pressure within the arteries which run in parallel with the contraction and relaxation of the heart. These waves create a continuous mechanical strain which goes on day in, day out without us noticing it – even at night when we sleep.

It is not surprising then that our arteries show some "wear and tear" as we grow older (A man or woman, it has been said, is as old as his/her arteries). This is due to the incessant mechanical strain and to many other factors. In the course of this inevitable ageing process our arteries thicken and develop "lesions" that bulge out more and more and in the end may hinder the flow of blood. To a certain extent this happens in all of us. By the time we are 30, visible changes in our blood vessels will have occurred – some people have more some have less, but nobody is entirely free of this process called arteriosclerosis. Thus cardiovascular diseases, mainly caused by *arteriosclerosis*, are by far the most frequent ailments. They are responsible for the premature death of more people than any other condition (Figure 1) and have therefore been rightly termed the No 1 KILLER in all industrialised countries.

Because the heart is such a vital organ, arteriosclerosis is most dramatically felt here – even though the same process occurs in other parts of the body as well. When the narrowing of a coronary artery exceeds a certain limit, the transport of blood and oxygen will be critically impeded. The result is a shortage of oxygen, particularly when demand for oxygen is high e.g. when the heart beats fast as during physical exercise or emotional stress. This lack of blood/oxygen is called ischaemia/hypoxia in medical terms and is felt as pain: angina pectoris as doctors call it. Characteristically this pain is felt in the heart, right arm or shoulder and is accompanied by intense anxiety and fear as well as difficulty in breathing.

A similar series of events can, of course, also happen in other arteries. If the arteries supplying the brain are affected, we will not typically experience pain but might feel a slight dizziness indicating that the nervous system cannot function properly due to lack of oxygen – in

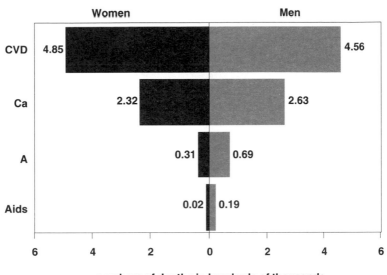

CVD = cardiovascular disease

Ca = cancer

A = accidents

Figure 1
Leading causes of death (USA 1989)

severe cases this can be much more dramatic and result in a stroke, the brain's equivalent of a heart attack. If the arteries of the legs are affected we will in the initial stages of the disease feel pain when we increase the demand for oxygen as during walking – doctors call this symptom intermittent claudication. As soon as such a patient stops walking the pain will ease off because the demand for oxygen decreases during rest. In later stages of peripheral vascular disease there may also be pain at rest and the leg might even become gangrenous.

Back to the heart; angina pectoris is often a warning signal. It should be taken very seriously indeed; with proper treatment we can slow down or even reverse the underlying process of arterial narrowing. If arterio-sclerosis continues, more and more ischaemia will ensue and one day a heart infarction might be the result.

A heart infarction or heart attack is caused by ischaemia so severe that a whole part of the heart muscle is virtually starved of oxygen. The affected heart muscle cells quite simply die as a result. Depending on how big the affected part is, the pumping function of the entire organ can or cannot continue. Most people nowadays survive such a heart attack not least thanks to significant advances in treatment, but many others will not live. In about one third of all cases a heart attack happens without the warning signal "pain", and death will then have been the first (and last) sign of coronary heart disease.

3 | The risk factor concept

The concept of risk factors may be best explained by giving an example. The suspicion that smoking causes lung cancer arose first through anecdotal evidence – it was noted that many smokers developed this disease. It needed large scale population studies to confirm this suspicion, and an association was firmly established. Finally intervention trials were required to make sure there was a cause–effect relationship, that smoking was in fact the cause of the cancer. These studies demonstrated that smoking cessation did significantly lower the incidence of cancer. Only with this type of evidence, can one be certain about a causal relationship and about the fact that smoking is a (causal) risk factor for lung cancer.

There are, of course, numerous pitfalls in such research. To take an exaggerated example, one might have noticed that most lung cancer patients have yellow fingers (from smoking). A strong association between the shade of yellow on the second and third finger of the right hand and the incidence of lung cancer could have been established. One might have contemplated viewing yellow fingers as a "risk factor" for cancer. Obviously this would have been wrong – not all associations, however strong, are causal in nature. An "intervention trial" would thus not have produced the anticipated result: bleaching the yellow fingers would obviously not have reduced the death rate of cancer.

To establish causality is therefore crucial; albeit difficult to do. Risk factors are defined as being causally related to the event under investigation, meaning they are somehow responsible for the result and represent (one of) the cause(s) of the problem.

This does not necessarily mean that there is a direct link nor that the disease has only one cause. Smoking may indirectly cause cancer, for instance through events that are triggered by one or more constituents of tobacco. Similarly smoking cessation will not prevent all lung cancers. There are more than one cause, and smoking is just one of them.

Thus the risk factor concept implies causality but not mono-causality of disease. Most diseases have many causes. Eliminating one risk factor will merely reduce the chances of this disease occurring, it can't solve the problem entirely. The concept of risk factors goes a long way in telling us something about probabilities; it does not predict with certainty what will happen to a given individual.

This concept is highly advanced in the area of cardiovascular disease. Some 50 years of intense research have helped to identify a substantial number of risk factors (Table 1). Some factors can be changed others can not; the latter ones are important only in as much as they tell us who is at particularly high risk. Potentially changeable risk factors can lead us to effective means of disease prevention.

4 | Which are the most important cardiovascular risk factors?

Blood lipids are on top of the list of risk factors for coronary heart disease. When research in this area started, cholesterol (often also termed total cholesterol) was at the centre of interest. Meanwhile we know that two subfractions of blood lipids are of particular importance: LDL (low density lipoprotein, 60-70% of the total cholesterol is transported in this fraction) and HDL (high density lipoprotein). The former is a major risk factor: the higher the LDL level, the more likely the problem of coronary heart disease. HDL on the other hand has some protective potential: the lower its level the higher the risk of heart disease.

Blood lipids like cholesterol are essential for numerous body functions. Only when they are not in balance do they become a real hazard to our health. In this case they are deposited in excess amounts within the arterial vessel wall and speed up this complicated chain of events which leads to arteriosclerosis (see Chapter 2). If arteriosclerosis affects the arteries that supply the heart itself, we call this coronary heart disease.

A strong, graded and positive association between total cholesterol and subsequent coronary heart disease has been observed so many times that there cannot be any dispute about its existence. There is no clear threshold level above which this risk becomes apparent, and the association is stronger in men than in women who, generally speaking, seem to be protected to a certain degree from coronary heart disease up to the time of menopause. In patients with established coronary heart disease the association becomes much stronger than in healthy individuals. Clinical trials in which cholesterol levels were lowered by diet or medication have shown that this reduces the number of heart attacks and deaths, both in apparently healthy individuals and those already affected by coronary heart disease. On average a 10% reduction of cholesterol leads to a 20% reduction of risk of coronary heart disease. Since these studies were usually short-term trials, the true effect might be even larger; some estimate it to be about 33%. There is also a dose-effect-relationship: the greater the cholesterol reduction the stronger the effect on the risk. Other studies have shown that the progression of *arteriosclerosis* (see Chapter 2) can be retarded by cholesterol reduction.

Blood lipids are affected by several other risk factors. For instance smoking, obesity, diabetes and physical activity may modify the lipid pattern. Usually the risk increases over-proportionally in individuals who are burdened with more than one risk factor: having, for instance, two risk factors more than doubles the threat.

In addition to total cholesterol, LDL and HDL there are other lipids which determine the risk, triglycerides and lipoprotein (a) are examples; their true importance is, however, still the subject of intensive debate.

It must be re-emphasised that our knowledge about risk factors in general and cholesterol in particular is very recent and therefore most likely incomplete. The first big population study started only in the late 1940's. It is a project that is still continuing. Amongst others it demonstrated that men and women with cholesterol levels higher than 275mg/decilitre (dl) are burdened with 3-10 times the risk of recurrent heart infarction and about twice the risk of death compared to those with cholesterol levels below 200mg/dl. Values between 200 and 220mg/dl may therefore well be what we should aim for.

Even though lipids are important, they are by no means the only risk factors for coronary heart disease (Table 1). *Diabetes*, both the type that needs insulin therapy and the one that can be treated without injections, is associated with an increased risk of coronary heart disease, particularly in women. How this risk is brought about is not yet fully understood; to some extent diabetes increases other risk factors but more direct mechanisms are also suspected. For diabetic patients it is essential to control the disease and the blood sugar level in the best possible way; this will also diminish the chances of falling victim to coronary heart disease or any of the other complications of diabetes.

Cigarette *smoking* is probably the most unhealthy habit of all. It causes various cancers and many other ailments. But most importantly it is a prominent risk factor for coronary heart disease. Even passive smoking (inhaling the smoke of others) is probably harmful, even though this is less well established. The effects of cigarettes on the circulation are multifold.

Amongst others, a constriction of the arteries and detrimental changes within the composition of the blood can be observed. The younger an individual smoker is, the more harmful smoking will be for him/her. On the other hand, when people manage to quit the habit (actually it is an addiction) the cardiovascular risk level quickly returns to normal. The message here is clear: the sooner you give up, the better.

Blood pressure is another important risk factor. Many studies have uniformly demonstrated that high blood pressure represents a high risk for coronary heart disease. Blood pressure can be lowered by a variety of means, e.g. diet, changes in life style and drugs. Lowering blood pressure has also been shown to reduce the risk of heart attacks and death.

A summary of all available data implied that a reduction of 5-6mm Hg diastolic blood pressure is followed by a 42% reduction of risk of stroke. In terms of risk of coronary heart disease, the evidence is less straight forward and still the subject of investigation and debate.

Physical inactivity is also strongly associated with the risk. Regular activity will affect other cardiovascular risk factors like lipids and blood pressure but it probably also has an independent effect. Physical activity is beneficial both for healthy individuals and for patients with coronary heart disease. In the latter group a well balanced exercise programme can reduce the death rate by 20-25%.

5 | Therapy and prevention

From the above discussion it follows that one should not focus on one but on all risk factors. In other words treat hypertension and diabetes *and* also give up smoking etc.

If you have elevated cholesterol levels, the first thing to try is a healthy diet preferably combined with a wisely planned exercise programme. Avoid fatty food, particularly those which contain plenty of animal fats. Eat more starchy food like vegetables and fruit. If you are overweight eat less altogether and normalise your weight. It is highly advisable to seek professional, individualised advice from your GP and possibly a dietician. Current thinking is that a Mediterranean diet with lots of pasta, vegetables, fruit, fish and olive oil is one of the best diets to prevent heart disease. Also it is now becoming more and more accepted that *moderate* use of (red) wine is beneficial.

Your doctor will also tell you about exercise. If you have been sedentary for years, don't start abruptly. Allow some time to become adapted and build up a routine that suits your physical fitness, your daily needs and that you enjoy. To have fun is important! If nothing else, it will make you stick to the newly altered life-style. Endurance exercises are much more suited than body building programmes. The best exercises are those where the whole body is active, e.g. walking, swimming, bicycling etc. Competitive sports like squash can be hazardous to the untrained individual; it is important to plan the activity wisely and to stop when it gets too much – this may be difficult in a competitive setting. Regularity is vital; exercising in a moderate fashion about three times a week will soon build up fitness. Subsequently you may do more and get more fun out of it.

In many cases a balanced diet combined with regular exercise will be sufficient to bring cholesterol levels into the safe range. If not, most doctors will prescribe lipid lowering drugs. There are several such drugs available today (Table 2). All of them are effective in reducing cholesterol. One disadvantage, however, is that they may cause side-effects.

Having elevated cholesterol levels is not a disease, it is a risk factor (see Chapter 3). People feel perfectly healthy even with exceedingly high levels. By being put on (life-long) medication with possible unpleasant side effects a healthy person is turned into a patient. Often patients will not tolerate this and just not take the prescribed drugs. Sometimes they tell their doctor, sometimes they don't.

The other factor to consider are costs; they can be substantial for drugs (Table 2). The challenge therefore is to find a remedy that lowers cholesterol but without ill effects, is accepted by the patient and is inexpensive. Garlic may be just that.

6 | Garlic as a herbal drug

Garlic has been used as a medicinal plant in (many if not) most cultures since antiquity. Yet it was only relatively recent investigation that clarified its constituents. The main ingredient is alliin which is contained at a concentration of about 10g/kg bulb. Alliin is a sulphur – containing compound but it is without smell. The typical odour of garlic is produced when the fresh garlic bulb is destroyed, and an enzyme (alliinase) breaks it down to alliciin. Alliciin in turn is degraded into ajoene and several polysulfides. The latter are responsible for the characteristic smell of garlic. The alliin content of the natural garlic varies by a factor of 10; decisive factors are the characteristics of the plant, soil and climate. Garlic also contains some carbohydrates and a large number of aminoacids and adenosine as well as substances with antibacterial activity like garlicin. .

One can, of course, take garlic pure in its fresh form. Cooking may destroy some of its activity and the amount required would put most people off (see below). Alternatively one may choose to buy commercial preparations of garlic. There are pills that contain dry garlic powder and capsules that contain oil macerates or volatile oil. The difference between the various formulations in terms of allicin content can be about 20-fold. Most of the recent clinical data has been obtained using a garlic powder pill. It is standardised to contain 1.3% alliin, which corresponds to an allicin release of 0.6%.

7 | The effects of garlic

Among the many hundreds of medicinal plants, garlic (latin name: allium sativum) is probably the one where the evidence for its usefulness is strongest. The medicinal use of this plant goes back to the stone age. Its first recorded mention dates back some four and a half thousand years! It was and is used in Europe, Russia, The Balkans, China, India and Egypt. Garlic is believed to originate from the Orient. In many civilisations it is used as a spice for cooking – a fact that may be important when discussing its safety (see below).

Research into this plant has been going on for decades and has become very acute during the last 10 years. The evidence is now scientifically so compelling, that, in Germany (where most of the recent research has been performed), a prescription drug based on garlic has been officially registered.

Early and compelling evidence for the cardioprotective effects of garlic comes from the so-called Seven Countries Study. In this investigation some 1200 men aged 40-59 living in seven different countries were initially examined and then observed for a period of 15 years. The highest rates of coronary heart disease were found in those countries where little garlic was consumed (i.e. Finland) while the "garlic eating nations" like the Mediterranean countries had a much lower risk. Such studies are very interesting in that they put researchers onto the right track. However, they can never provide proof or disproof, simply because too many other factors, from genetic make-up to lifestyle variables, may play an important role and could have produced spurious findings.

Garlic has many beneficial effects that help protect our heart, but the most prominent and important medicinal effect of garlic is that of normalising blood lipids. Compared to some new, powerful synthetic drugs, the effect may be less pronounced. Yet, for most individuals a combination of garlic, diet and exercise will bring the cholesterol levels into the normal range.

In the course of the development of arteriosclerosis, blood lipids are oxidised which makes them even more dangerous. This process is inhibited by the anti–oxidant activity of garlic which significantly adds to its lipid lowering potential.

At present it is not entirely clear how exactly the lipid effects are achieved. The majority of the evidence indicates that the production of cholesterol, that takes place in the liver, is inhibited in the presence of the constituents of garlic.

The true attraction of garlic is that it has a number of additional effects that may help prevent coronary heart disease. As detailed above, high blood pressure and diabetes are other risk factors. Garlic significantly lowers mildly elevated blood pressure, and there is some evidence that it normalises blood glucose levels in diabetic patients. It also improves *blood flow* by making blood more fluid and blood cells less sticky as well as platelets less aggregable. Furthermore garlic has been shown to influence the *clotting* system of the blood in such a way that thromboses are less likely to form and more likely to be dissolved if they did cause an obstruction.

Garlic also protects the heart in more direct ways. It was shown that it prevents irregular heart beats and injury of the cells when there is a

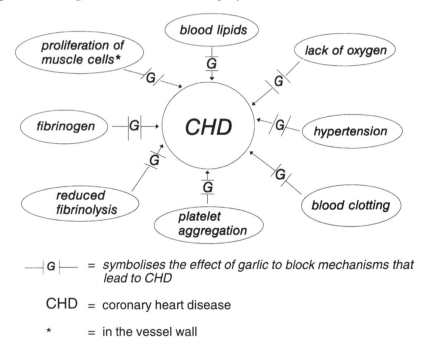

—| G |— = symbolises the effect of garlic to block mechanisms that lead to CHD

CHD = coronary heart disease

* = in the vessel wall

Figure 2

shortage of oxygen. Finally it limits the ability of the cells in the vessel wall to grow, multiply and form an obstructing arteriosclerotic lesion; such effects can be demonstrated for instance in cell-cultures.

The multitude of these effects may work synergistically in the prevention of coronary heart disease (Figure 2). Even if each effect in itself may be weaker than that achievable by other powerful synthetic medications, it is this multifactorial potential of garlic that renders it a highly promising treatment. To phrase it differently: in order to obtain all the beneficial effects that garlic produces, one would need to take an awful lot of synthetic drugs.

Some effects are potentially useful for other diseases most of which have been demonstrated in animal models or test tubes (Table 4). Garlic has been shown to kill bacteria, viruses and fungi and to stimulate the immune system which renders it potentially useful for treating infection or even cancer. Experiments have also demonstrated that garlic inhibits tumour growth. Whether this can be used for the prevention of cancer needs to be investigated in more detail.

8 | Results from medical research

One of the first controlled clinical trials on patients with high cholesterol levels was conducted in the early 80's by our own research group. We investigated 20 such patients who were given either a cholesterol-lowering diet or the diet plus pills containing 600mg dried garlic powder per day. Figure 3 shows the changes in blood lipids observed after 12 and 24 days of treatment. Cholesterol, triglycerides and LDL were all lowered by garlic medication.

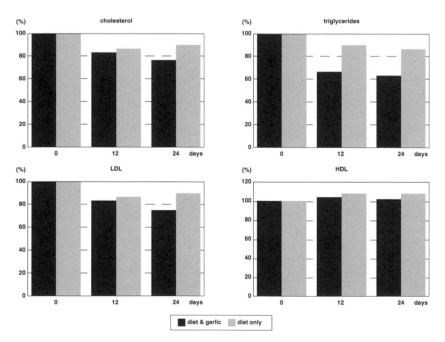

Figure 3
Changes in blood lipids with garlic treatment

The cholesterol-lowering effects have been confirmed repeatedly by various researchers in trials that were larger and methodologically more sound than ours (Figure 4). The action of garlic on triglycerides has also been reproduced many times. The effects are strikingly similar to the ones on cholesterol (Figure 5).

% change from baseline

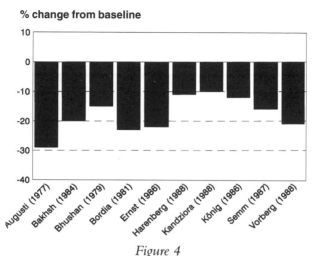

Figure 4
Results of some clinical trials on the effects of garlic on cholesterol

% change from baseline

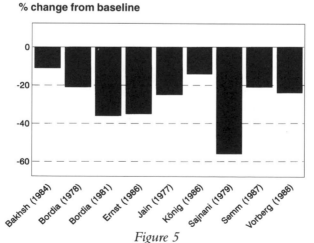

Figure 5
Results of some clinical trials on the effects of garlic on triglycerides

The cumulative data from all randomised controlled trials published to date (16 studies) imply that the medication with garlic will lower cholesterol by 0.77mmol/l more than an inert placebo pill. Again compared to placebo, triglycerides were lowered by 0-31mmol/l (Table 3). A similar analysis of the published literature concluded that the average decrease attributable to garlic medication was 0.6mmol/l which is equivalent to a fall of 9%.

A relatively recent trial is particularly illuminating. In this study, conducted by Mader in Germany, more than 200 patients with elevated cholesterol levels were treated either with placebo or with garlic pills. The results (Figure 6) demonstrate an average decrease of cholesterol of 12% and of triglycerides of 17%. If cholesterol was extremely high to start with, this effect was even more pronounced.

Other researchers investigated whether garlic would alter the dramatic increase in triglycerides that is usually seen after a fatty meal. For this purpose health volunteers ate two test meals with no less than 100g butter. In one instance they had been pre-medicated with 900mg garlic powder, in the other no pre-medication was given. The rise in triglyceride was markedly attenuated when garlic had been given.

Our own group has tested whether garlic also lowers cholesterol when it was not elevated to begin with. This study on normal volunteers demonstrated a decrease of total cholesterol levels even in these

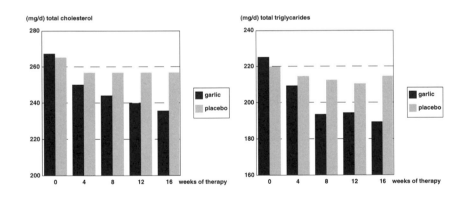

(according to Mader FH 1991)

Figure 6
The effects of garlic on cholesterol and triglycerides in a large sample
of patients with elevated cholesterol levels

individuals. As expected, the drop was less than in patients with elevated levels but it was nevertheless significant and clinically meaningful.

In most studies garlic is compared to placebo, and there can be no question that it is superior to such a dummy pill. But does it lower cholesterol as efficiently as a standard medication? One trial investigated this issue by comparing garlic with bezafibrate, the most commonly used lipid-lowering drug in the UK. The results were highly encouraging: in both groups cholesterol fell by about 25%. So garlic can be as effective as the medication prescribed by your GP, but it may, of course, have advantages in terms of side-effects (see below).

Obviously it matters for how long the garlic is taken; the effect on cholesterol grows with time. The data from all relevant studies pooled together (Figure 7) implies that the maximal effect is reached after 3 months. There are not enough studies with medication-periods longer than this, but there is no reason to assume that the effect wears off after 3 months.

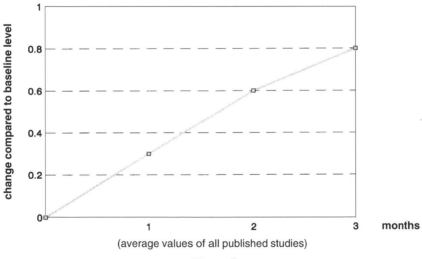

Figure 7
Effects of cholesterol over time

Figure 8 summarises the results of studies on blood pressure. Six such studies have been conducted against placebo, on more than 400 patients altogether. The medication of garlic is superior to placebo in lowering both systolic (during heart contraction) and diastolic (during heart relaxation) blood pressure. Again the effect is more pronounced if blood pressure was elevated to start with. Therefore garlic may be of some clinical use in subjects with mild hypertension. As this condition is a very important risk factor for cardiovascular diseases (see above), particularly stroke, garlic might be a useful preventive measure for individuals at risk. The fibrinolytic activity of blood is important in preventing blood from clotting. A blood clot is also called thrombosis and is a major element in the events immediately before most heart infarctions. There are several studies demonstrating that garlic has beneficial effects in this respect.

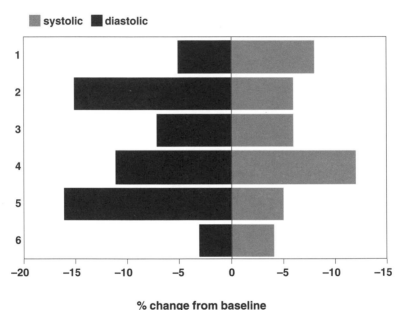

% change from baseline

1 Harenberg (1988)
2 Kandziora (1988)
3 König (986)
4 multicentre trial (1988)
5 Petkov (1966)
6 Vorberg (1988)

Figure 8
Results of some clinical trials of the blood presure of garlic

These trials are summarised in Figure 9. Most of them show a very marked enhancement of fibrinolytic activity implying that garlic can prevent thrombosis which may cause an infarct.

Most clinical trials also agree that the administration of garlic inhibits platelet aggregation. This must be viewed as a positive effect, since platelet aggregation is a key phenomenon leading to the complex changes on and in the vascular wall which eventually bring about arteriosclerosis and coronary heart disease.

Other studies show that patients' fluidity of blood can be enhanced through the medication of garlic. This leads to a better flow of blood even in the most tiny capillaries. Similarly this was accompanied by a small degree of vasodilatation which means an enlargement of blood vessels again contributing to better flow.

One recent study demonstrated that patients given garlic pills exhibited an enhanced metabolic control of glucose. These individuals experienced a 12% reduction in blood glucose levels, which was significantly more

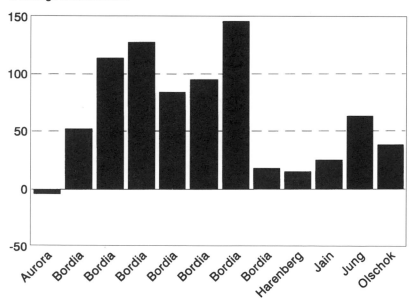

Figure 9
Results of some clinical trials on the effects of garlic on fibrinolytic activity

than in those patients that were treated with a dummy pill. These effects might be important for diabetics, but we need more research in this particular area.

Finally the anti-oxidant capacity mentioned above has also been demonstrated clinically. After patients had been given 600mg garlic powder for 2 weeks, a 34% reduction in the susceptibility of lipoproteins to oxidation was noted. This effect is considered meaningful because it prevents oxidation in the body and oxidised lipoproteins may exert particular harmful effects and promote arteriosclerosis.

9 | Are there side-effects?

Herbal remedies are often assumed to be entirely safe. This is a dangerous misunderstanding. Like all oral drugs, herbs may cause problems and the possibility of side-effects needs serious consideration. In fact there is no reason to assume that the receptors in our body can discriminate between synthetic and natural compounds. Therefore a chemical from a plant can do as much harm as one from a factory. Herbalists claim that, because plants contain a variety of compounds, there can be a synergy in terms of the desired effect. This claim is at present only poorly substantiated; it should be stressed that a synergy, should it exist, could work towards desired as well as adverse effects. Thus herbal remedies are associated with an under-researched and complex safety issue.

Plants that have a long tradition are likely (but not guaranteed) to be safe as any problem, it may be assumed, would have appeared a long time ago. Herbs that are traditionally used in food, like garlic, are particularly likely to be safe; because of the frequency of their use, adverse reactions would have shown up and be well known by now. *Yet there are no guarantees; to be entirely sure one needs proper tests.*

In the case of garlic, this has been done and the results are re-assuring indeed. A minority of individuals may develop gastrointestinal symptoms, like (mild) nausea, but this usually only happens when the recommended dose of garlic has been exceeded significantly. Occasionally there can also be allergic reactions. Otherwise garlic is completely safe, even for long-term use. The trial data show roughly the same frequency and severity of side-effects as with placebo. One could not possibly wish for a better safety record! The typical odour may be a disadvantage for some. My advice is to persuade your partner to consume garlic as well – then he/she won't mind.

10 | Who should take garlic?

In Germany the authorities have licensed garlic for the following indications:
- assistance of dietary treatment of elevated blood lipids
- prophylaxis of age-related changes in the circulation

The latter indication, it seems, would render a large proportion of the general population potential users of garlic.

There are two different strategies in disease prevention. Firstly one can target the whole population. One might, for instance, aim at reducing cholesterol levels of an entire nation – say by modifications of the diet. Secondly one might prefer to identify a sub-group that is at a particular risk and modify the risk only in these individuals. Both approaches have their strengths and weaknesses: targeting the whole population might be potentially more beneficial in terms of lives prolonged but it also might be unreasonably expensive or just not acceptable to the majority and therefore doomed to failure. On the other hand, targeting high risk sub-groups might be of limited overall effect albeit affordable.

In the case of prevention of coronary heart disease, it is an accepted fact that individuals with extreme values of one risk factor (e.g. particularly high cholesterol and/or blood pressure) will respond particularly well to a given intervention (see above). Therefore prevention in this area might be best targeted to these people. Following this line of thought, three groups of individuals should take prevention particularly seriously:
a. patients with established vascular diseases
b. individuals burdened with one or more risk factors
c. close relatives of individuals belonging to either group a. or b.

To confine prevention to those three groups would, however, be wrong. As garlic represents a relatively cheap and harmless form of treatment, anyone who feels strongly about the issue should consider it. My advice is that he or she discusses the pros and cons with a physician who is well informed about prevention in general and garlic in particular.

11 | Which dosage?

On the basis of the published evidence, it is difficult to provide definitive recommendations as to the optimal dosage. Most of the clinical trials have been conducted with garlic powder pills. Three times 300mg/day seems to be a dosage which produces the desired effects. Fresh garlic is variable in terms of content of allicin. Therefore the dosage can vary from half to one clove per day; on average a daily dose of 4g fresh garlic will suffice.

12 | Conclusions

Garlic has stood the "test of time". It is a very safe and effective means of positively influencing accepted risk factors of coronary heart disease. It can therefore help protect the heart from arteriosclerosis. Its most notable effects are a normalisation of the lipid profile of the blood. Garlic has been tested extensively in animals, volunteers and patients. It has considerable potential in the prevention of cardiovascular disease and death.

13 | Further reading

This book has been written (mainly) for an interested lay audience. This often meant that complex issues had to be presented in a simple fashion. A little simplification, it has been said, saves tons of explanation. Yet the basic information in this book is accurate, true and complete.

Many readers might feel that they would like to learn more. To satisfy this need for detailed texts, the following reading list of relevant reviews is provided. Original work can be identified by searching the reference lists of these articles.

Block E. *The chemistry of garlic and onions*. Sci American 1985;252:114-19

E Ernst. *Cardiovascular effects of garlic*. Pharmather. 1987;5:83-9

Kleijnen J et al. *Garlic, onions and cardiovascular risk factors*. Br J Pharmacol 1989;28:535-44

Neil A, Silagy Ch. *Garlic, its cardio-protective properties*. Curr Opin Lipidol 1994;5:6-10

NN. *Prevention of coronary heart disease*. J Roy Coll Phys 1976;10:1-63

NN. *Strategies for the prevention of coronary heart disease*. Europ Heart J 1987;8:77-88

Pyorala K et al. *Prevention of coronary heart disease in clinical practice*. Europ Heart J 1994;15:1300-31

Reuter HD. *Allium sativum and allium ursicum Part 1 and 2*. Phytomedicine 1995;2:(Vol 1 and 2)

Silagy ChA, Neil AW. *A meta-analysis of the effect of garlic on blood pressure*. J Hypertension 1994;12:463-68

Silagy ChA, Neil AW. *Garlic as a lipid lowering agent - a meta-analysis*. J Roy Coll Phys 1994;28:39-45

Turner M. *Garlic and circulatory disorders*. J RSH 1990;3:90-93

Warshafsky S et al. *Effect of Garlic on total serum cholesterol. A meta-analysis*. Ann Int Med 1993;119:599-605

14 | Tables

Table 1
Accepted risk factors for coronary heart disease (CHD)

- Increased total plasma cholesterol
- Increased Low Density Lipo-Protein (LDL)
- Decreased HDL cholesterol
- Personal history of CHD
- Family history of CHD
- Cigarette smoking
- Obesity
- Male gender
- Hypertension
- Diabetes
- History of other cardiovascular disease, e.g. peripheral vascular disease

Table 2
Costs of lipid lowering interventions

Intervention	Amount per day	Effect on cholesterol	Annual Costs
COMA diet	35% energy as fat	12% ↓	none
Low fat diet	30% energy as fat	20% ↓	none
Cholestyramine (a)	3-6 sachets/day	20% ↓	£600
Bezafibrate	400mg/day	20% ↓	£120
HMGCoA reductase Inhibitor (b)	variable	30-40% ↓	£400
a+b combined	variable	40-50%	£1000
Garlic	600-900 mg/day (dried) or 10-20g (fresh)	~15%	

Table 3
Effects of garlic on blood lipids

Lipid fraction	mean change (%) beyond the effect of placebo
total cholesterol	−0.77mmol/1(12%)
triglycerides	−0.31mmol/l
LDL	
HDL	− no significant effect

Table 4
Effects of garlic that have been shown in the laboratory

Effect	Possible significance
Alteration of arachidonic acid metabolism	Arackidonic acid is a key compound determining a host of vascular functions
Antiarrhythmic effects	Stabilise the heart beat
Antibacterial activity	Self evident
Antifungal activity	Self evident
Antitoxic effects	Protection of vital organs like the liver or the heart from damage caused by toxins
Antitumor effects	Prevent cancer
Antiviral activity	self evident
Detoxification effect	Prevent organ damage from heavy metal intoxication
Inhibition of platelet aggregation	Platelet aggregate at the artery wall, a phenomenon that favours the arteriosclerotic process in a complex manner
Radical scavenging	"Free radicals" are compounds that can damage cells – garlic can neutralise these
Reduction in blood pressure	Blood pressure is a cardiovascular risk factor in its own right

OTHER AMBERWOOD HEALTH TITLES INCLUDE:

Aromatherapy – A Guide for Home Use by Christine Westwood. All you need to know about essential oils and using them. £1.99.

Aromatherapy – For Stress Management by Christine Westwood. Covering the use of essential oils for everyday stress-related problems. £2.99.

Aromatherapy – For Healthy Legs and Feet by Christine Westwood. A comprehensive guide to the use of essential oils for the treatment of legs and feet, including illustrated massage instructions. £2.99.

Plant Medicine – A Guide for Home Use by Charlotte Mitchell MNIMH. A guide to home use giving an insight into the wonderful healing qualities of plants. £2.99.

Woman Medicine – Vitex Agnus Castus by Simon Mills MA, FNIMH. The wonderful story of the herb that has been used for centuries in the treatment of women's problems. £2.99.

Ancient Medicine – Ginkgo Biloba by Dr Desmond Corrigan BSc(Pharms), MA, Phd, FLS, FPSI. Improved memory, circulation and concentration are associated in this book with medicine from this fascinating tree. £2.99.

Indian Medicine – The Immune System by Desmond Corrigan BSc(Pharms), MA, Phd, FLS, FPSI. An intriguing account of the history and science of the plant called Echinacea and its power to influence the immune system. £2.99.

Herbal First Aid by Andrew Chevallier BA, MNIMH. A beautifully clear reference book of natural remedies and general first aid in the home. £2.99.

Natural Taste – Herbal Teas, A Guide for Home Use by Andrew Chevallier BA, MNIMH. This beautifully illustrated book contains a comprehensive compendium of Herbal Teas giving information on how to make it, its benefits, history and folklore. £2.99.

Signs & Symptoms of Vitamin Deficiency by Dr Leonard Mervyn BSc, PhD, C.Chem, FRCS. A home guide for self diagnosis which explains and assesses Vitamin Therapy for the prevention of a wide variety of diseases and illnesses. £2.99.

Causes & Prevention of Vitamin Deficiency by Dr Leonard Mervyn BSc, PhD, C.Chem, FRCS. A home guide to the Vitamin content of foods and the depletion caused by cooking, storage and processing. It includes advice for those whose needs are increased due to lifestyle, illness etc. £2.99.

Eyecare Eyewear – For Better Vision by Mark Rossi Bsc, MBCO. A complete guide to eyecare and eyewear including an assessment of the types of spectacles and contact lenses available and the latest corrective surgical procedures. £3.99.